MENOPAUSE COUNTRY!

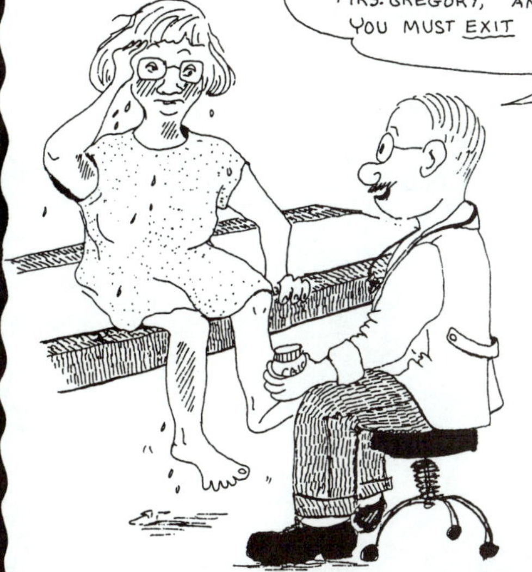

BY: JEAN ADAIR & HELEN GREGORY

MENOPAUSE COUNTRY
by
Jean Adair & Helen Gregory

Published by: Pinstripe Publishing   SAN 666-2889
   P.O.Box 711, Sedro-Woolley, WA 98284 USA

ISBN 0-941973-13-1

Manufactured in the
United States of America
10 9 8 7 6 5 4 3 2

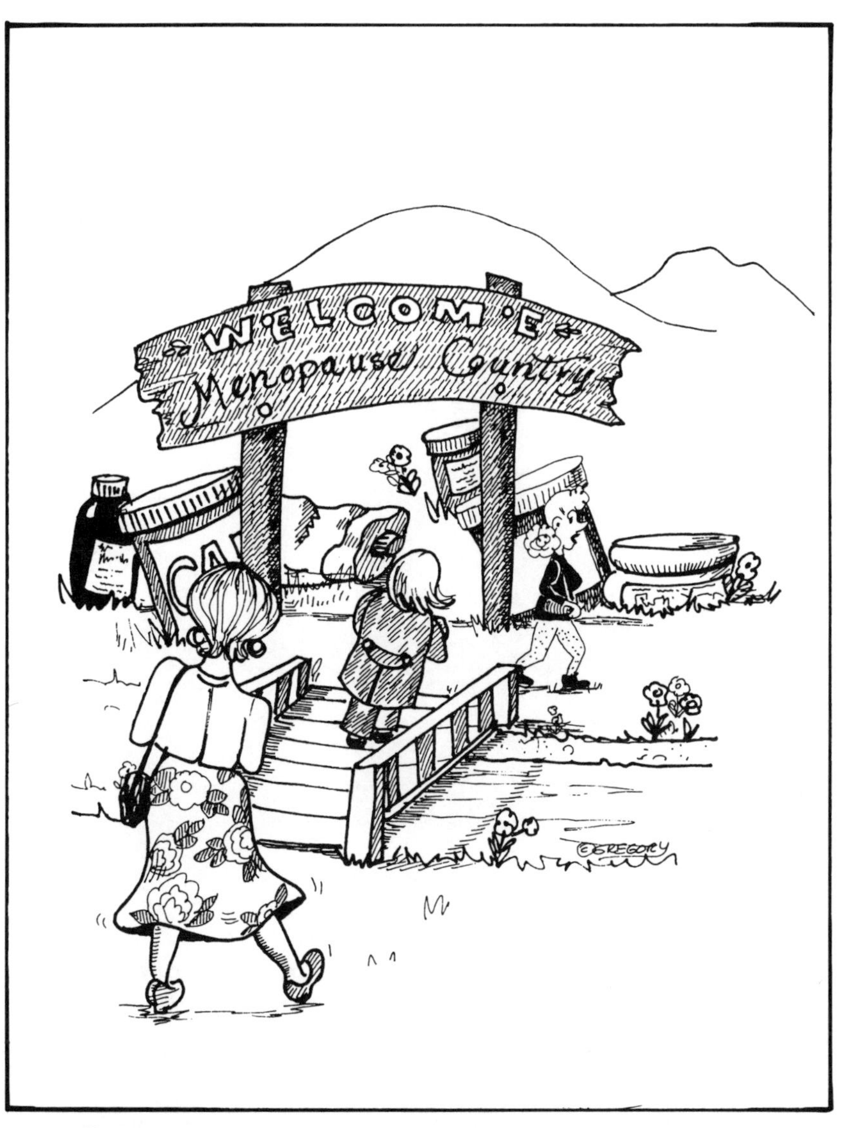

Baby boomers are just starting to enter menopause. For the first time, they have something in common with their mothers!

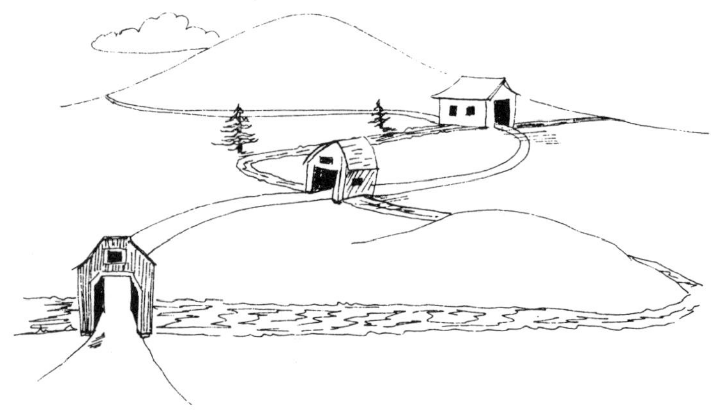

DEDICATION
*With understanding and loving humor, we
dedicate this book to our world-wide sisters
whose hormones (and various other body parts)
have gone south for the winter of our lives.*

Jean & Helen

The Bridges
of
Menopause Country

The Bridges of Menopause Country —
We approach them with panicky fright.
There's a feeling of dread
As they loom up ahead
And Clint Eastwood is nowhere in sight.

The Bridges of Menopause Country
Are not on the main tourist track.
You're just passing through,
Snap a photo or two,
Then learn that you cannot go back.

The Bridges of Menopause Country
Where the waters are roiling with foam,
Set your face!   Cut your loss!
Walk firmly across!
And come out, at last, safe at home!

C H A N G E S

Oh for days pre-menopausal
When life was "of course" and not "maybe"
When a PATCH was a place to pick berries
And CHANGE meant a clean diaper for baby.

When a HOT FLASH was just an announcement
That set all the news wires humming
And a PILL didn't bring back your girlhood,
It just kept more babies from coming.

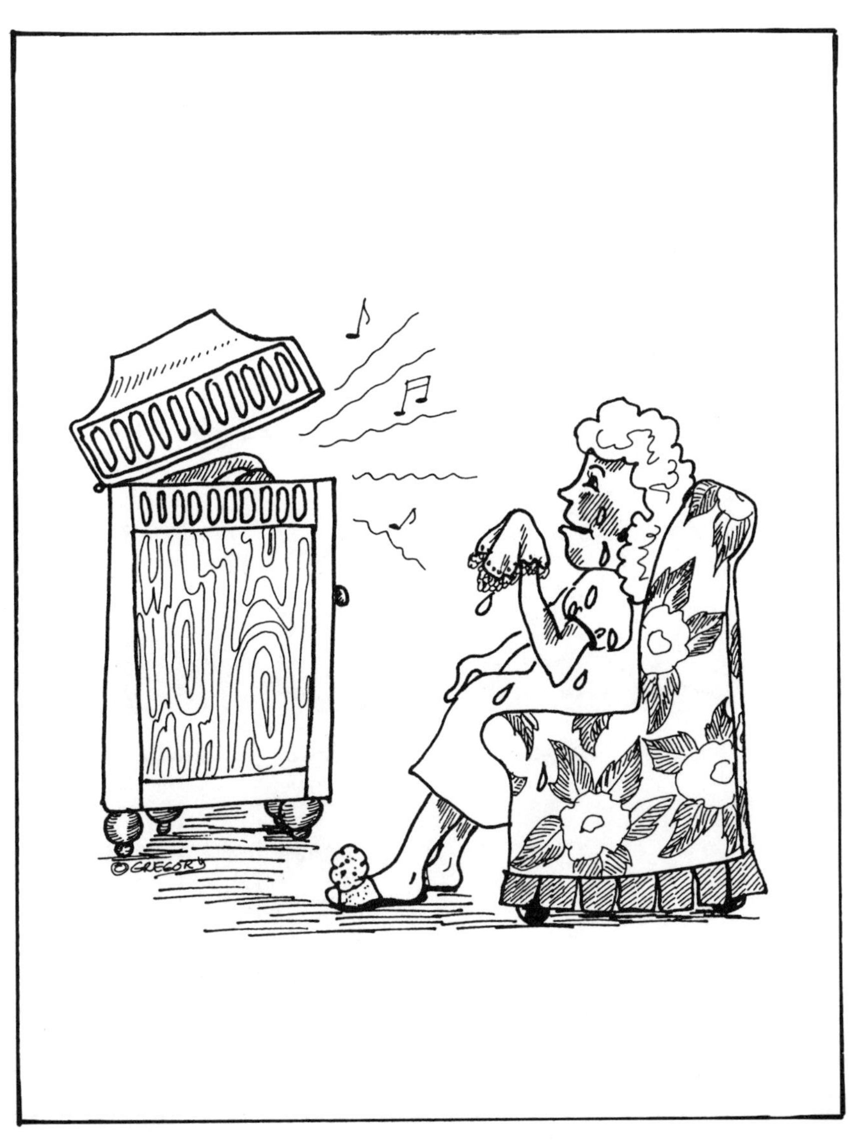

Menopause is when "Sweatin' to the Oldies" is a way of life, not a work-out tape.

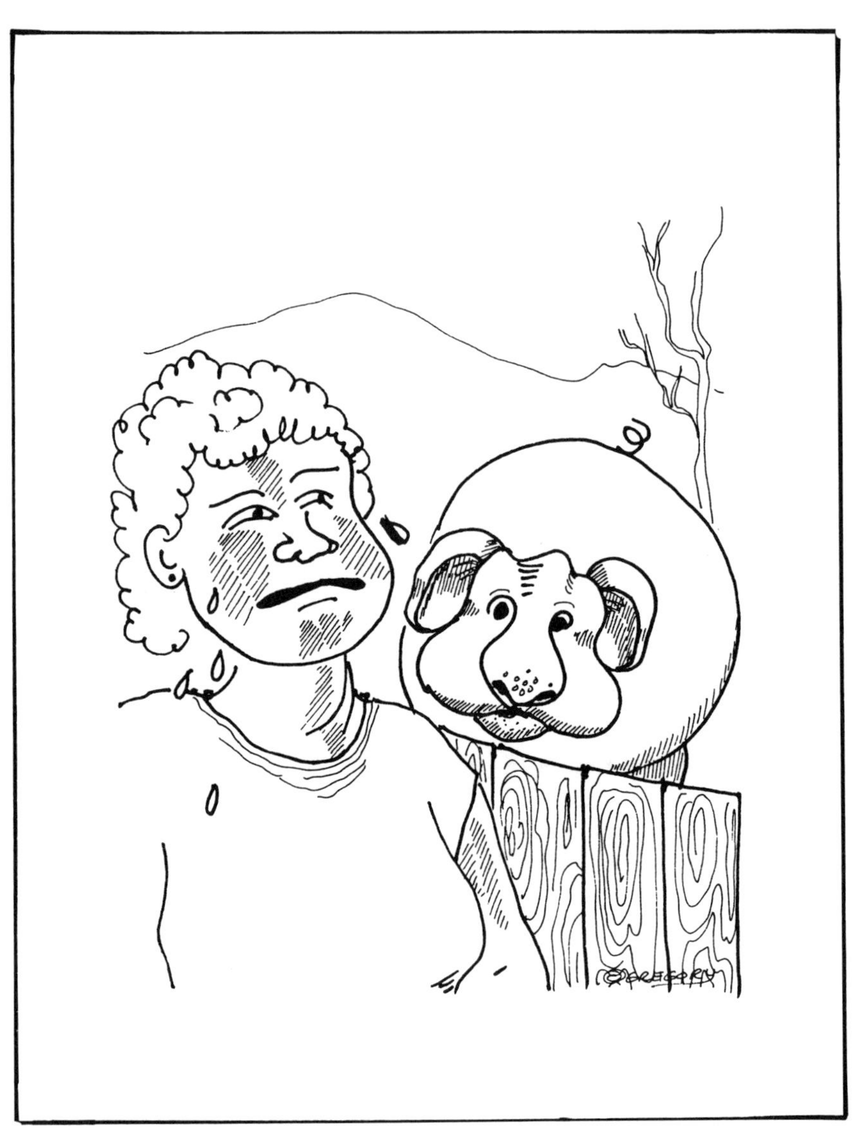

Menopause is when you learn that a
hypothalamus is not a zoo attraction.

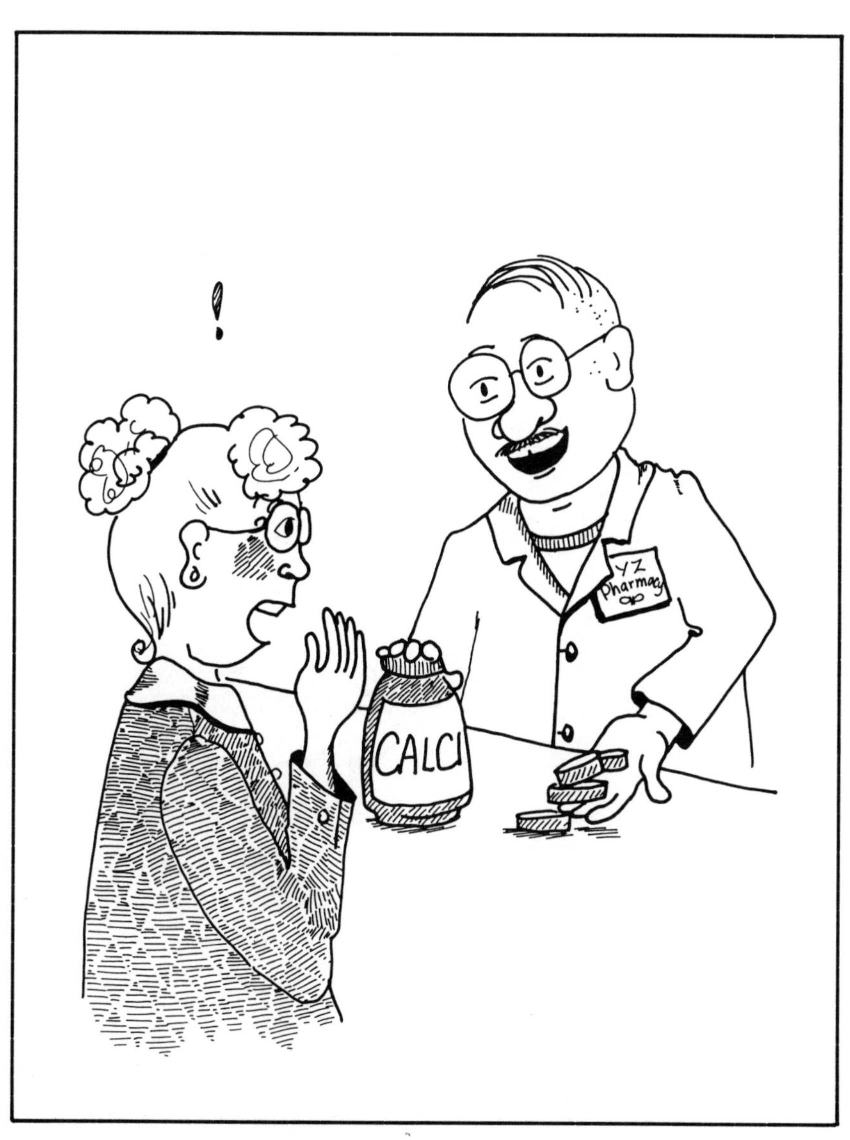

"*Just swallow four of these a day
with a sip of water.*"

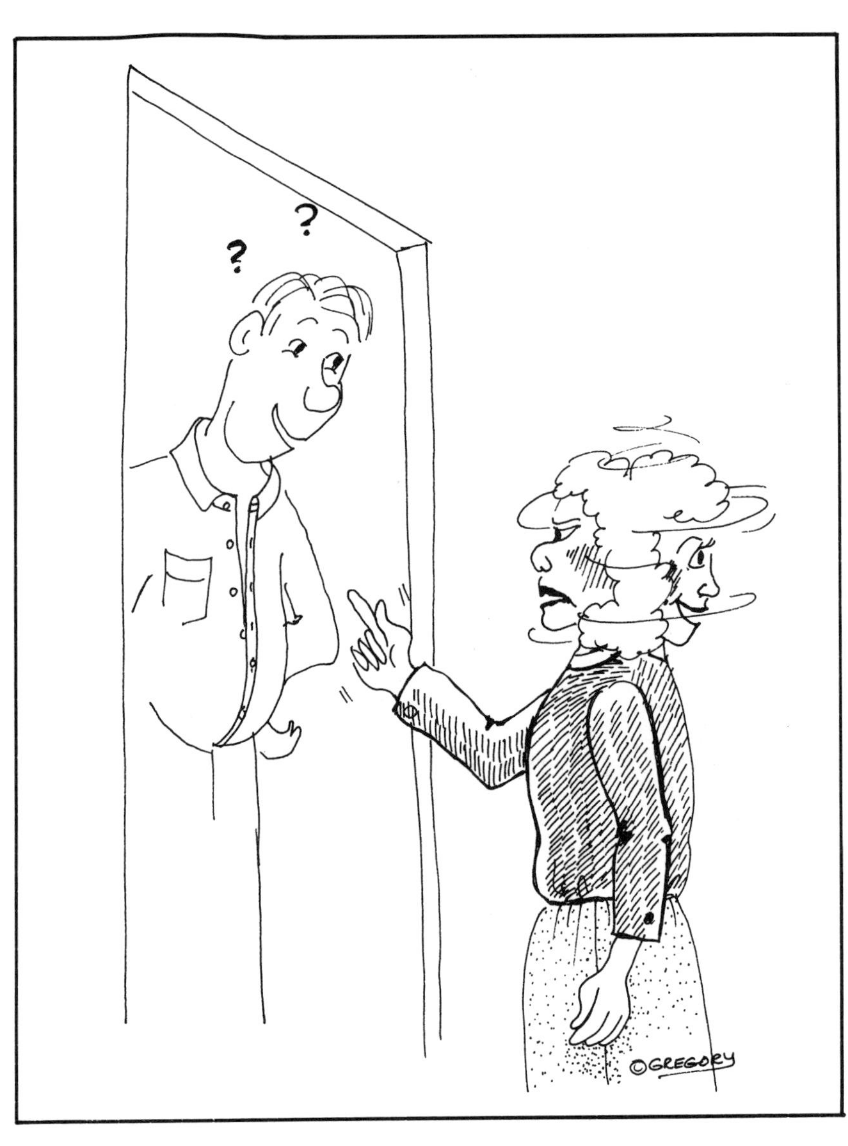

"No Dear, I don't think I have mood swings...
And I'll kill anybody who says I do!"

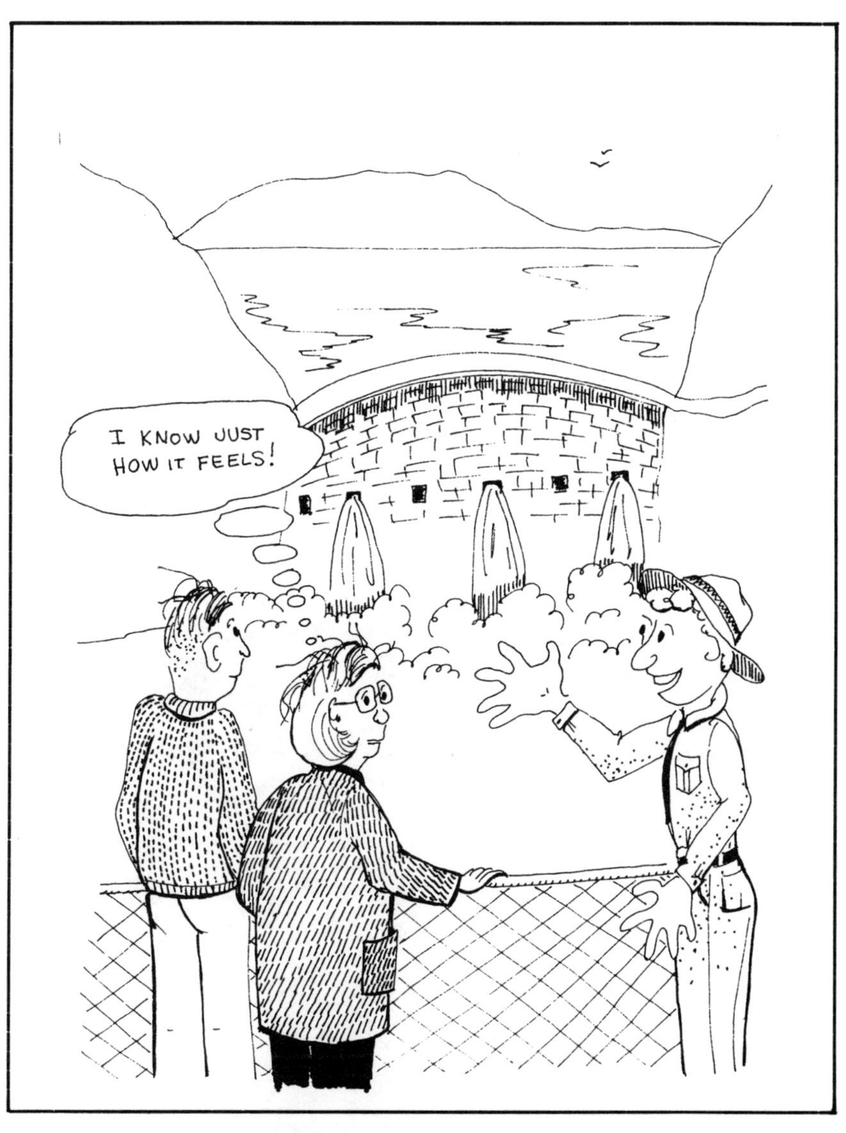

"This dam retains a total of 12 million cubic feet of water per day."

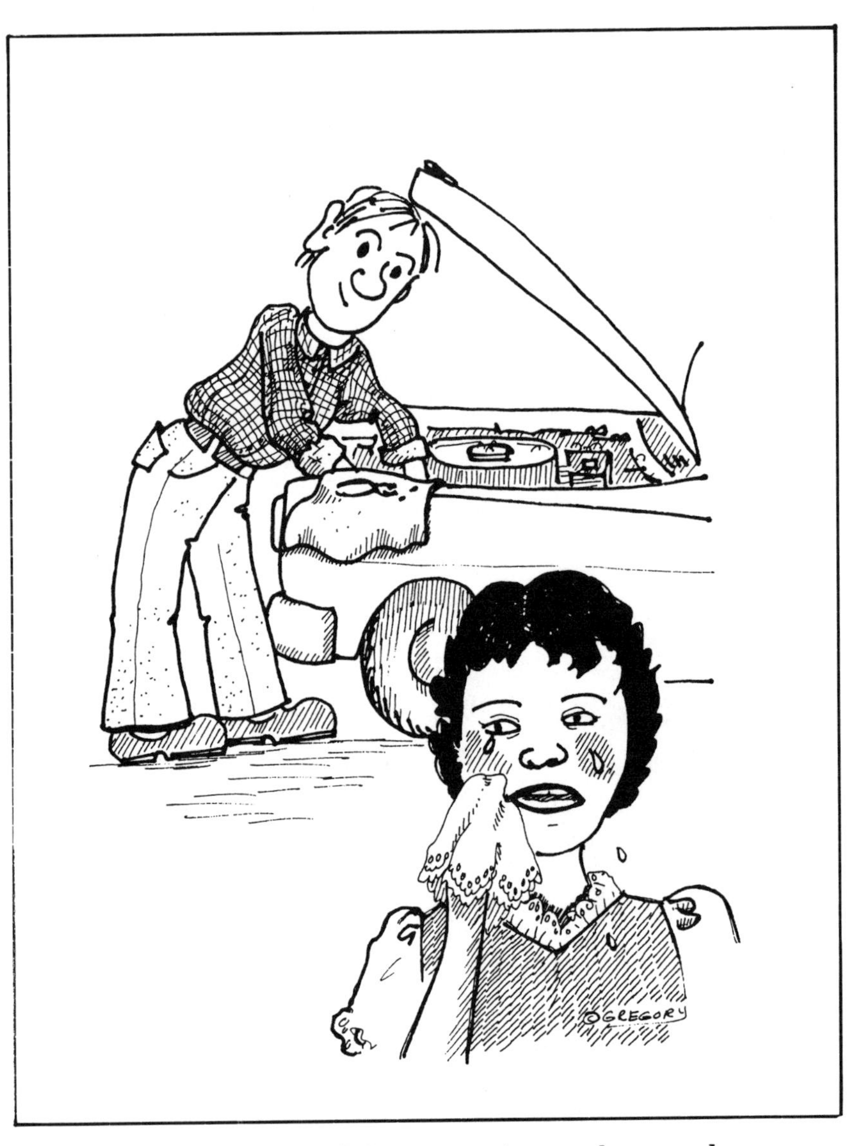

"Just because I have an irregular cycle,
it doesn't mean my timing gear is off."

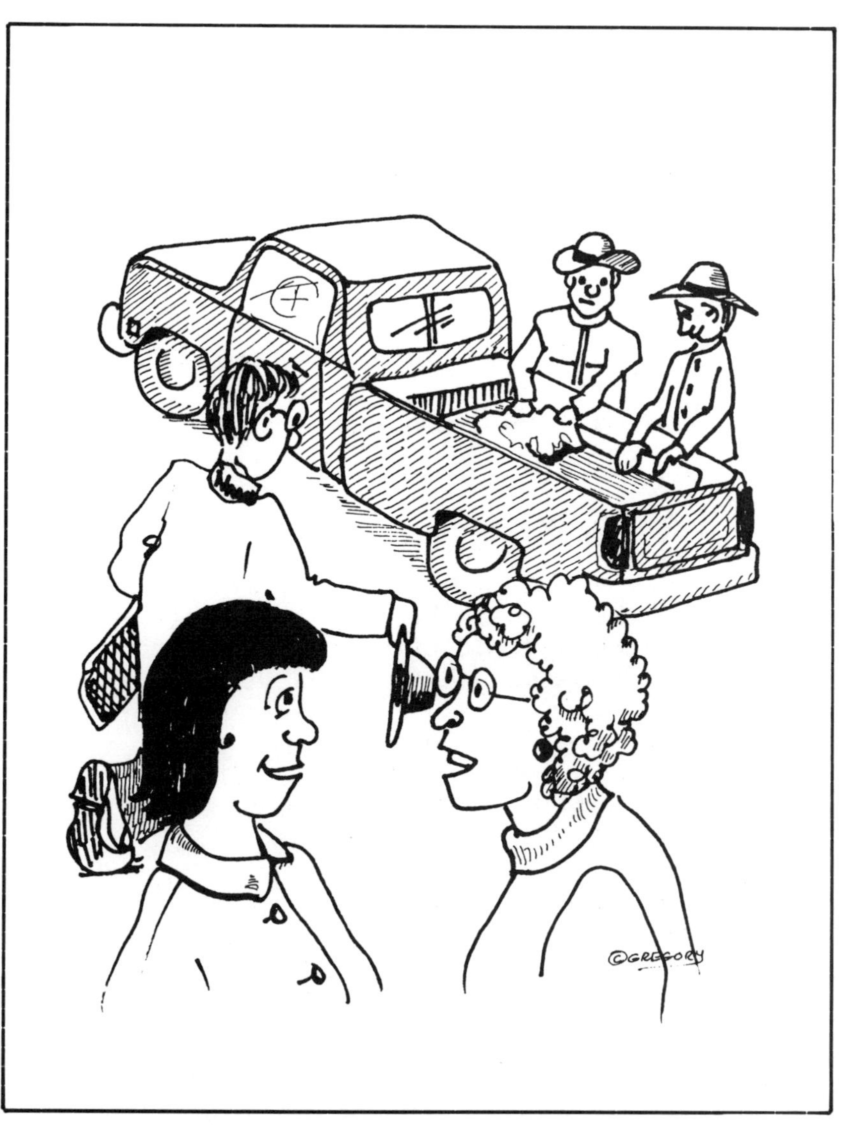

"Men go through the change of life annually.
They call it hunting season."

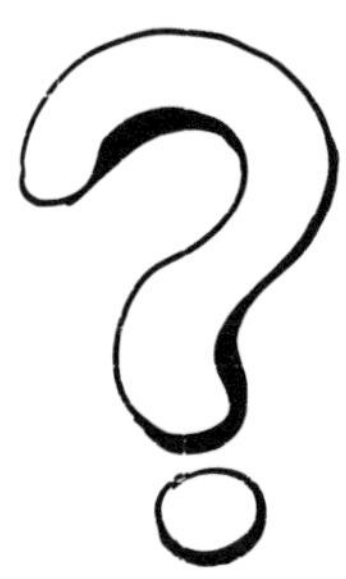

THE ESTROGEN QUESTION

Estrogen Replacement Therapy —
Debates rage hot!
Our ranks divide, as we decide
To ERT or not.

They say it causes (slows, prevents)
(fill in diseases here __________).
The hottest fad, for good or bad,
On drugstore shelves this year!

It can, it can't, it may, it might,
If often does (and will),
It should be bought (or maybe not)
As cream, or patch, or pill.

When doctors disagree, it's true:
We can't do much about it.
Where will we be with ERT?
What will we be without it?

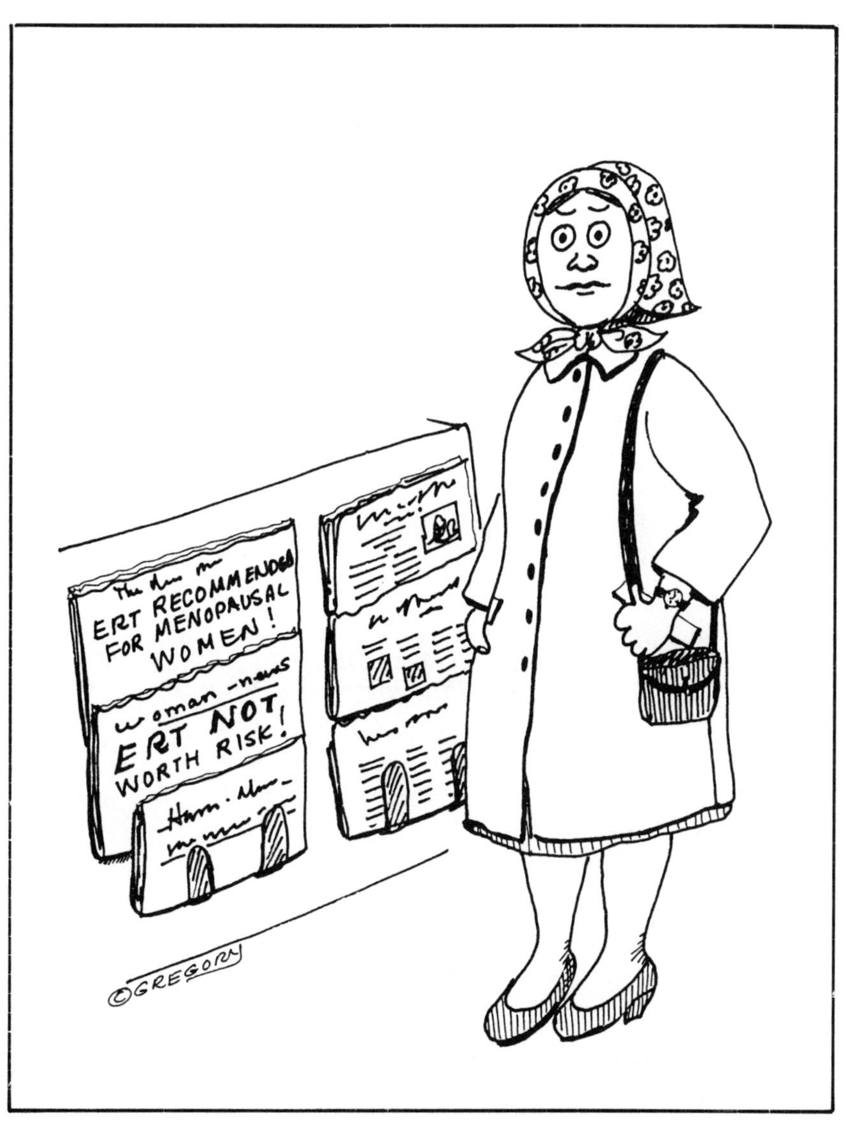

Mental confusion may be a symtom of menopause.

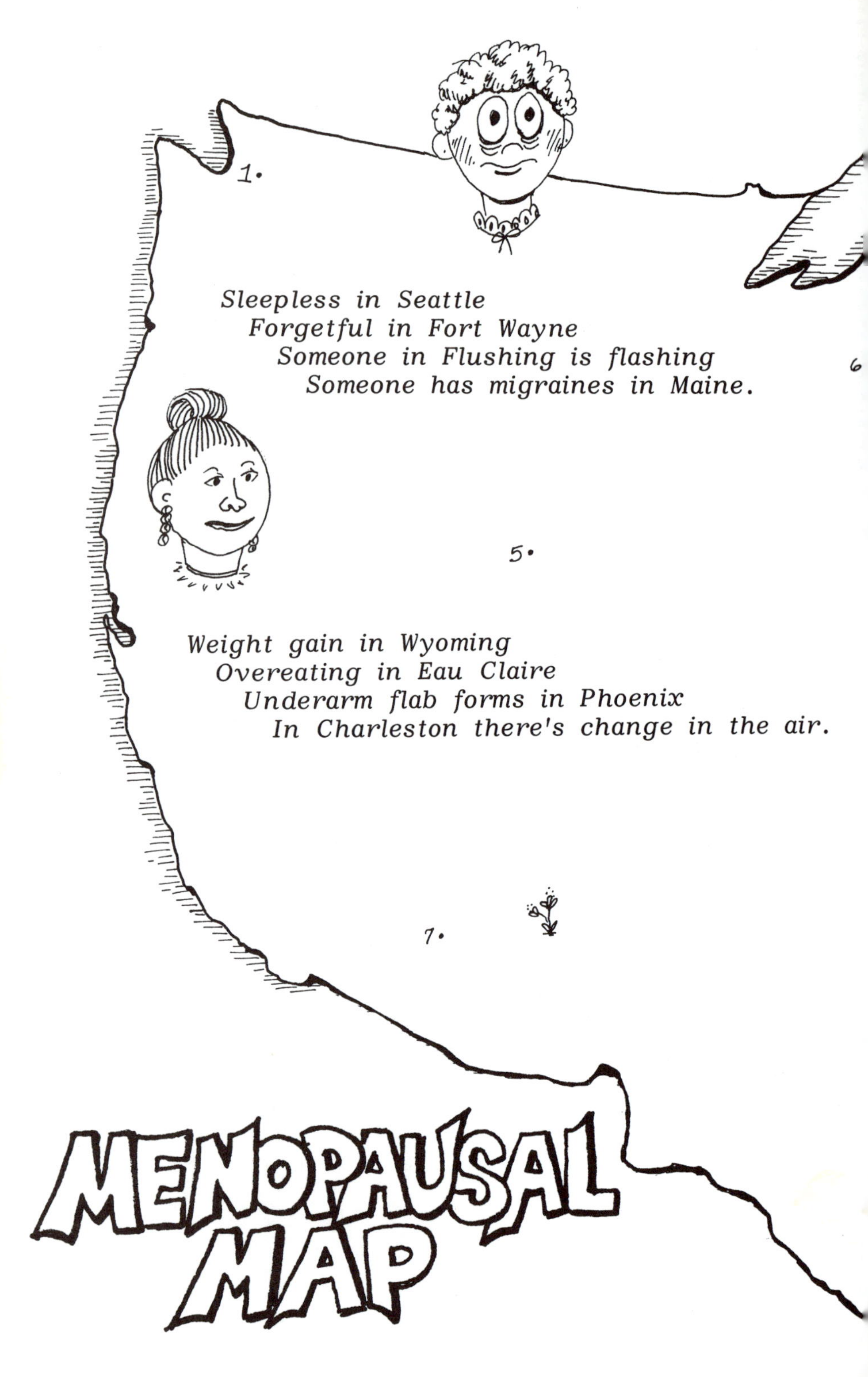

Sleepless in Seattle
Forgetful in Fort Wayne
Someone in Flushing is flashing
Someone has migraines in Maine.

Weight gain in Wyoming
Overeating in Eau Claire
Underarm flab forms in Phoenix
In Charleston there's change in the air.

MENOPAUSAL MAP

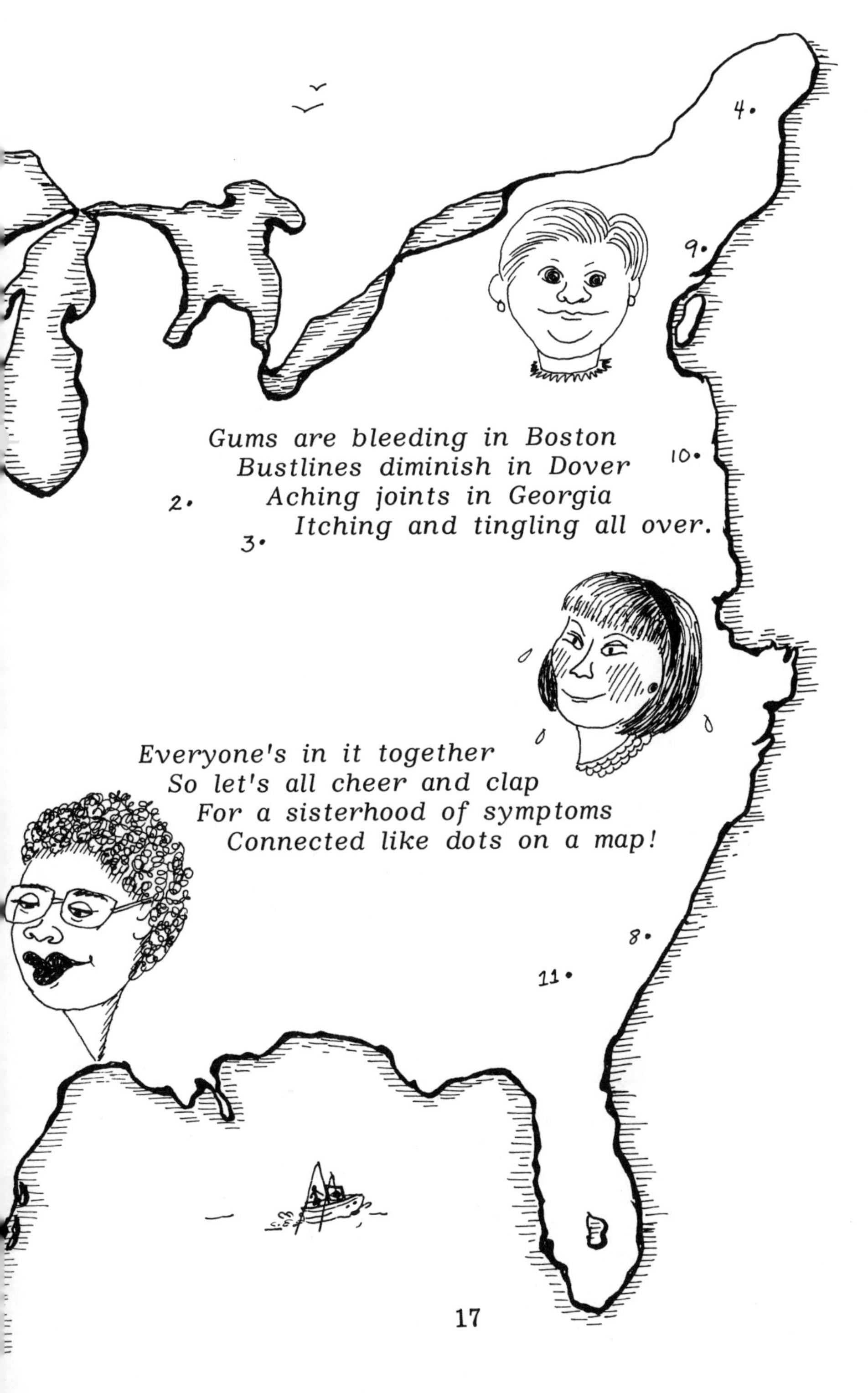
4.
9.
Gums are bleeding in Boston
Bustlines diminish in Dover
10.
Aching joints in Georgia
2.
Itching and tingling all over.
3.
Everyone's in it together
So let's all cheer and clap
For a sisterhood of symptoms
Connected like dots on a map!
8.
11.

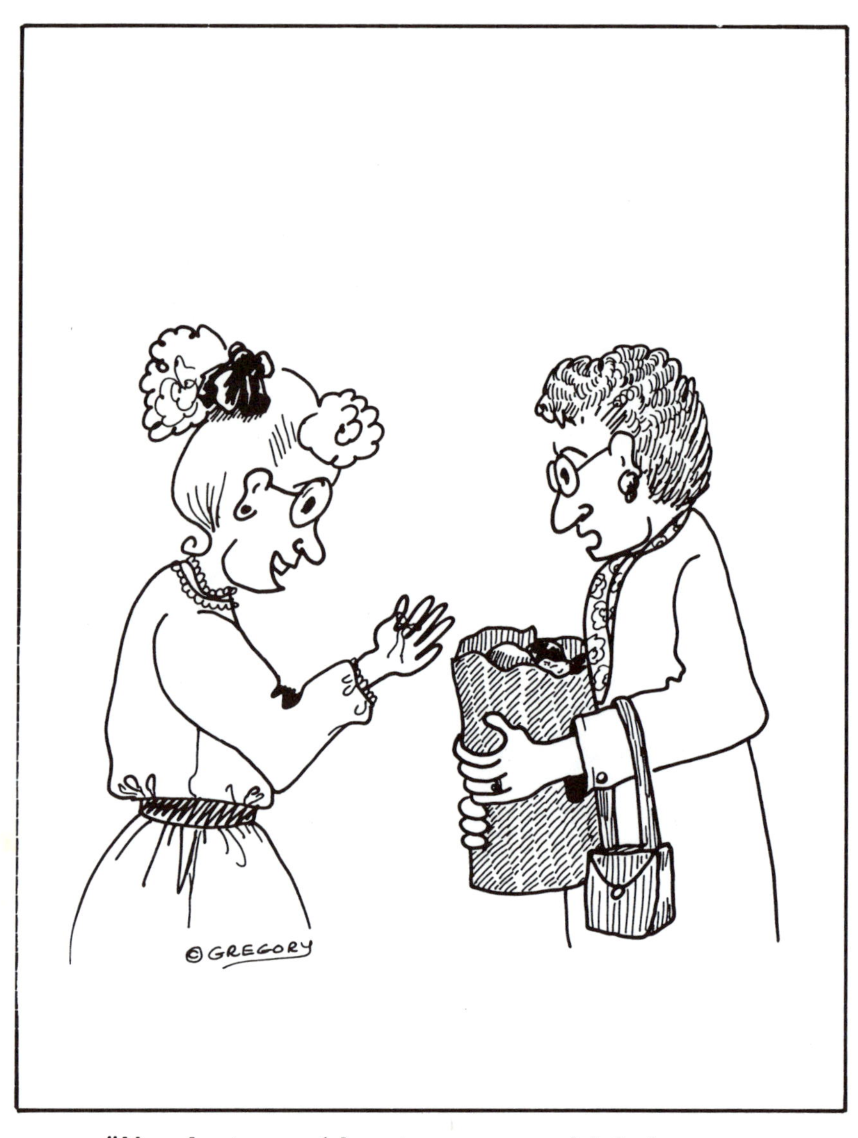

"My doctor said estrogen would help
with my memory loss.   Now, if I could
just remember to take it!"

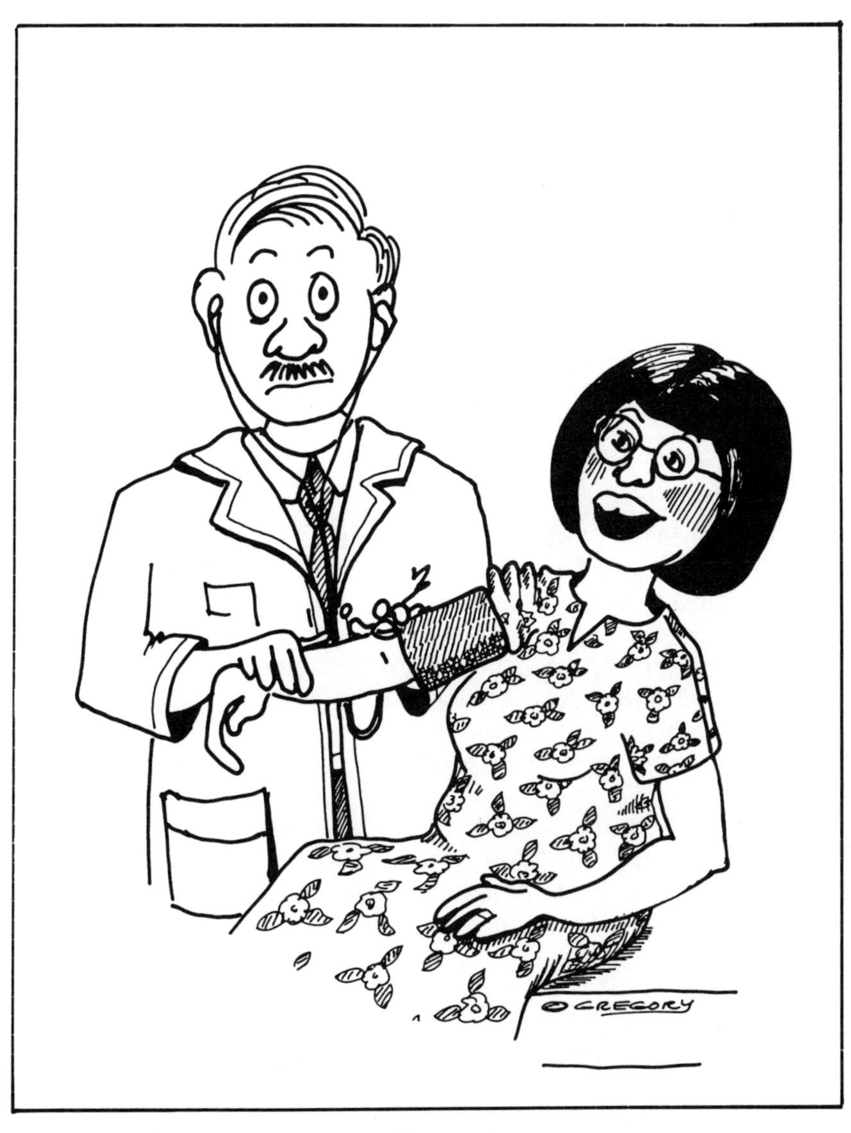

"Well, yes, little things DO upset me —
I break a nail, the mail is late, my husband
decides to spend a weekend with
his secretary..."

I'M NOT READY!

I'm not ready for menopause
I think I'll take a pass,
I just got quits with cramps and zitz
And coming late to class!

I haven't time for menopause
My kids are youngsters still.
Just 'cause they've grown kids of their own
I'm NOT over the hill!

I'm not prepared for menopause
For blowing hot and cold
Why, just last week I hit my peak...
How come now I'm old?

I'm not really ready for menopause
As anyone can see
But if my age is any gauge,
Menopause is ready for me!

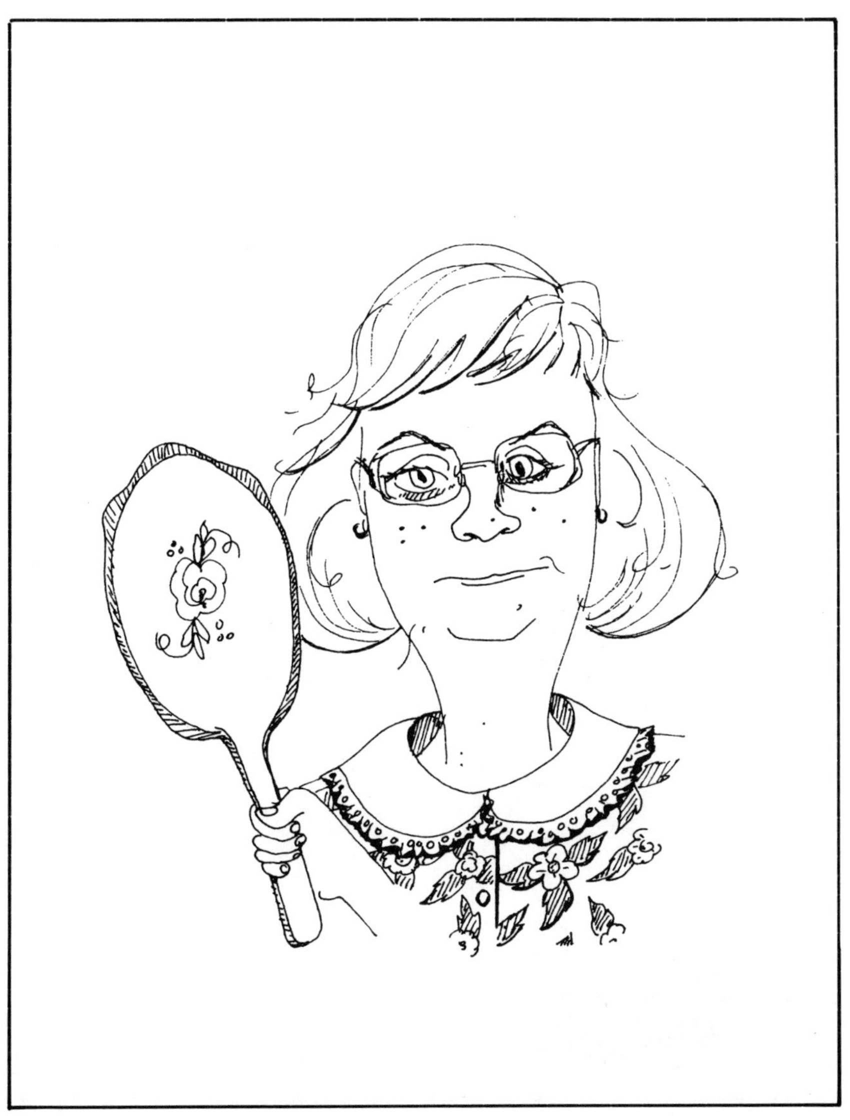

WHAT'S HAPPENING?

First you freeze and then you're sweatin'
Your body feels so new and strange.
Emotions storm and pimples threaten...
Puppy Love? No, just the change!

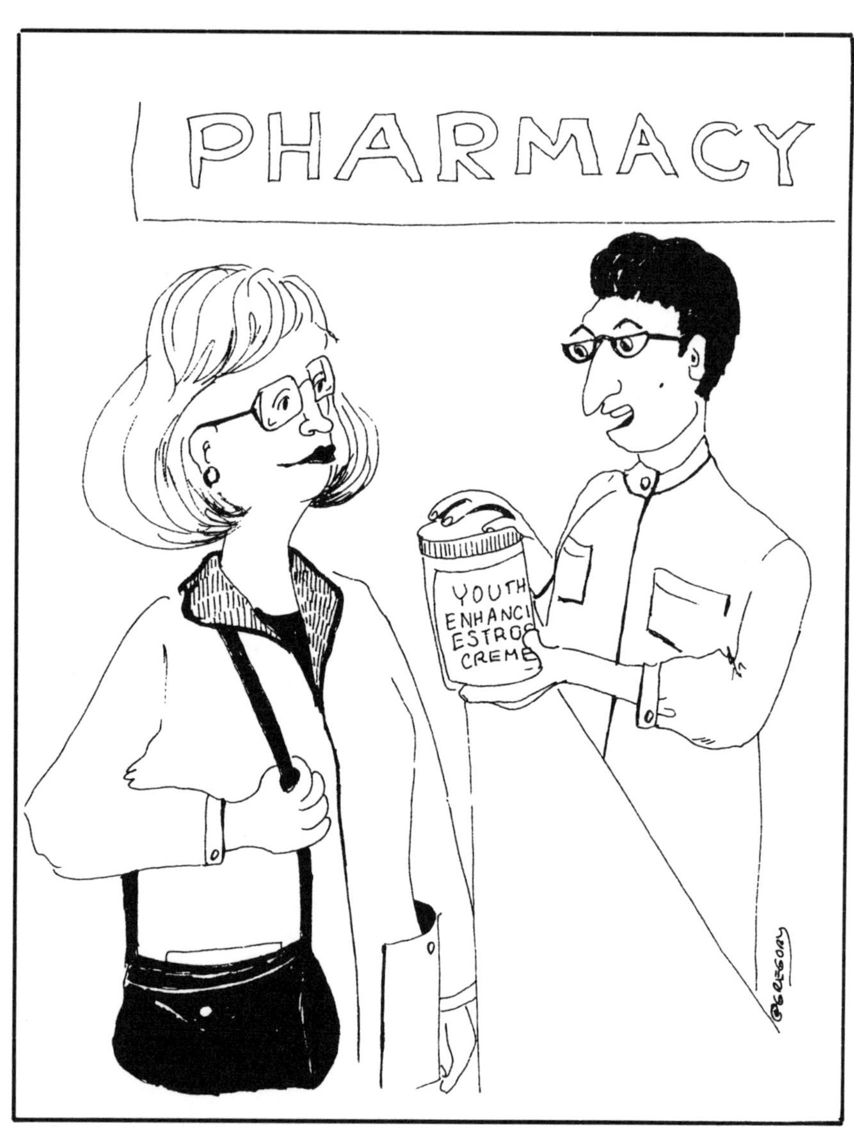

"Of course it can work miracles.
It got on the market, didn't it?"

CERTAIN AGES

"A woman of a certain age."
A fuzzy, half-formed phrase,
A euphemistic yardstick
For measuring our days.

It conjures frail ladies
Draped in shawls of lace
Fluttering fans, and moving
At a genteel pace.

Let's regard that "certain age"
As life's last phase and best;
Enjoy what Margaret Mead has called
"Postmenopausal zest."

The only other choice we have
As we reach that stage,
Is to be a woman
Of an "uncertain" age.

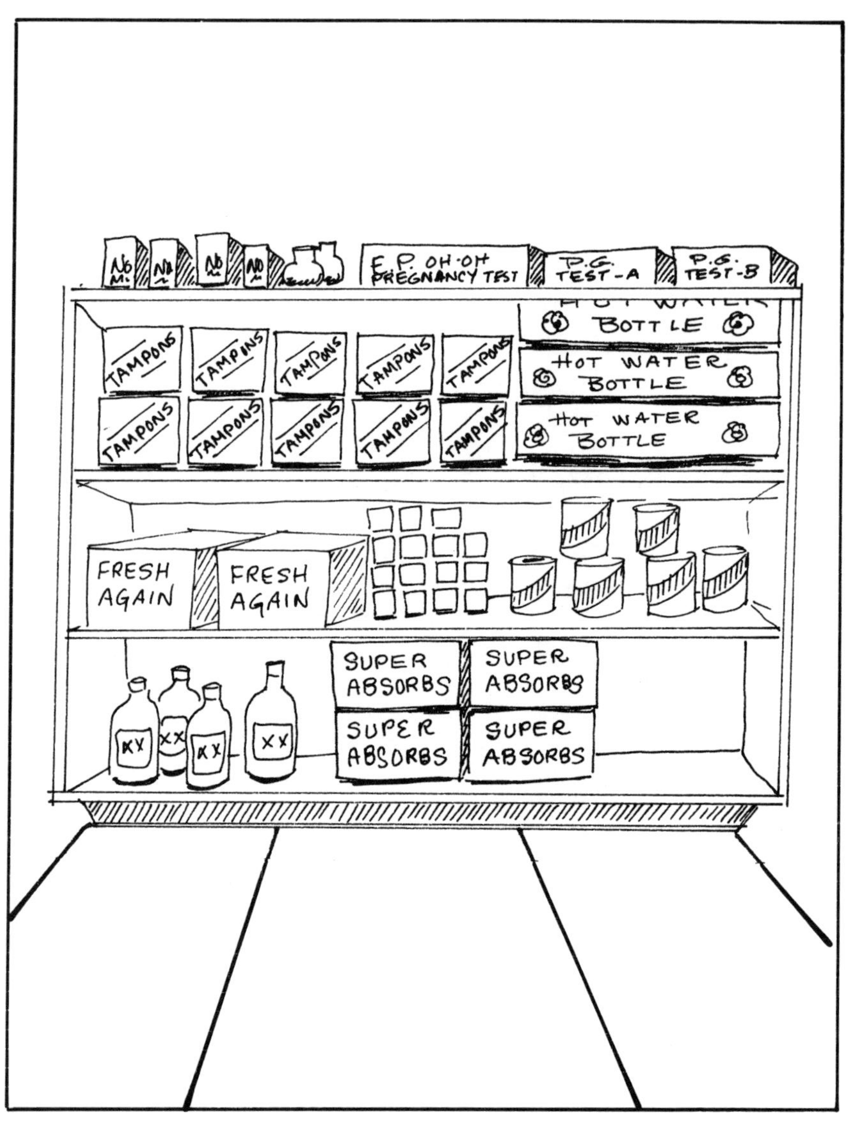

Drug store section most popular with pre-menopausal women.

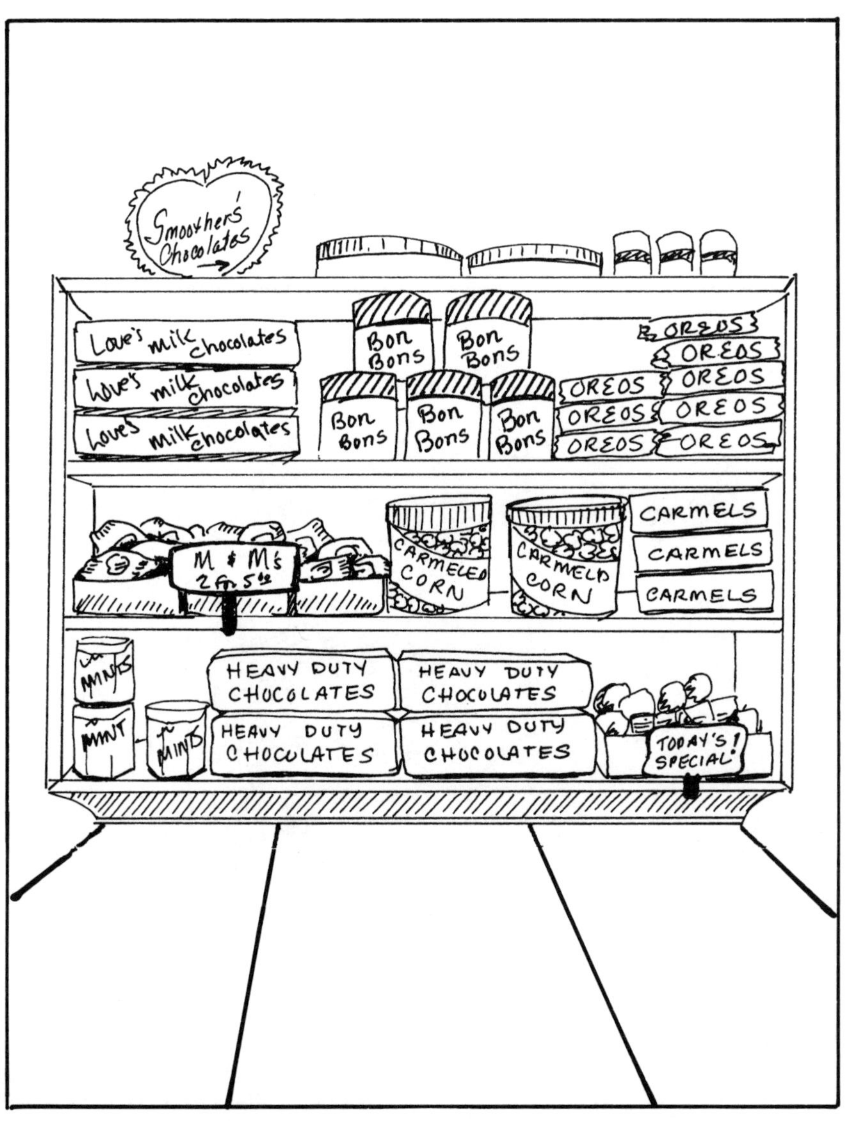

Drug store section most popular with menopausal women.

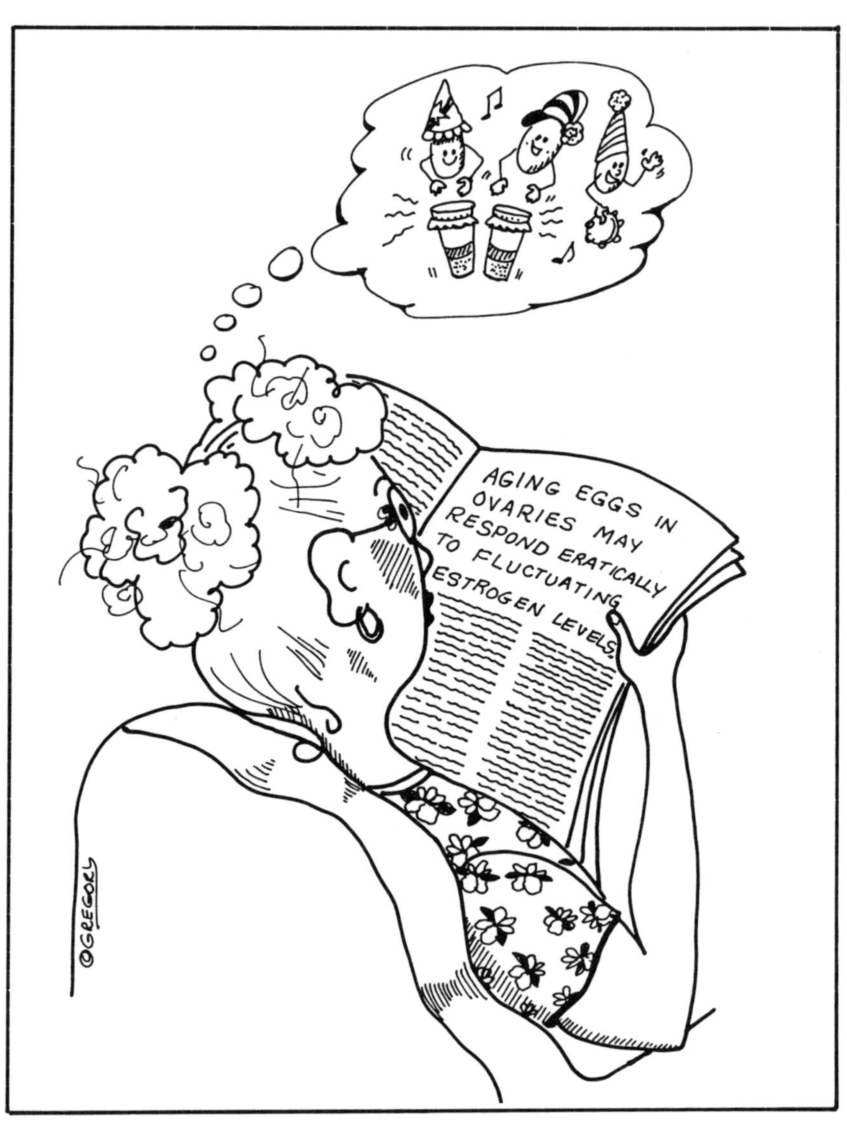

AGING EGGS IN OVARIES MAY RESPOND ERATICALLY TO FLUCTUATING ESTROGEN LEVELS.

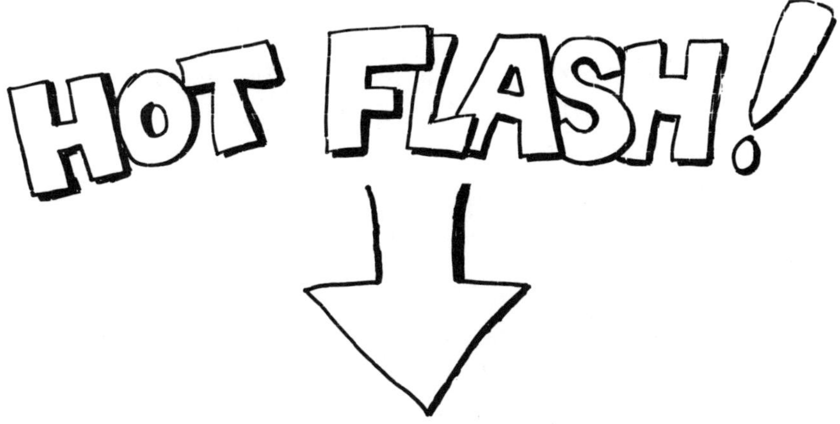

Estrogen can restore youth.
But who wants to go back to a
midnight curfew and wondering what
to wear to the prom?

10 REASONS TO ENJOY MENOPAUSE
(Well, 8 of them!)

1. You'll save large amounts of money
   on heating bills.

2. Memory loss means you won't remember
   what life was like before menopause.

3. You learn that fat cells produce a form
   of estrogen — at last they're good
   for something!

4. Hershey's!

5. Nestle's!

6. Cadbury!

7. You'll be able to work "estrogen," "progestin,"
   and "perimenopause" into the same sentence!

8. You'll be able to say: "Not this year... I've
   got a headache!"

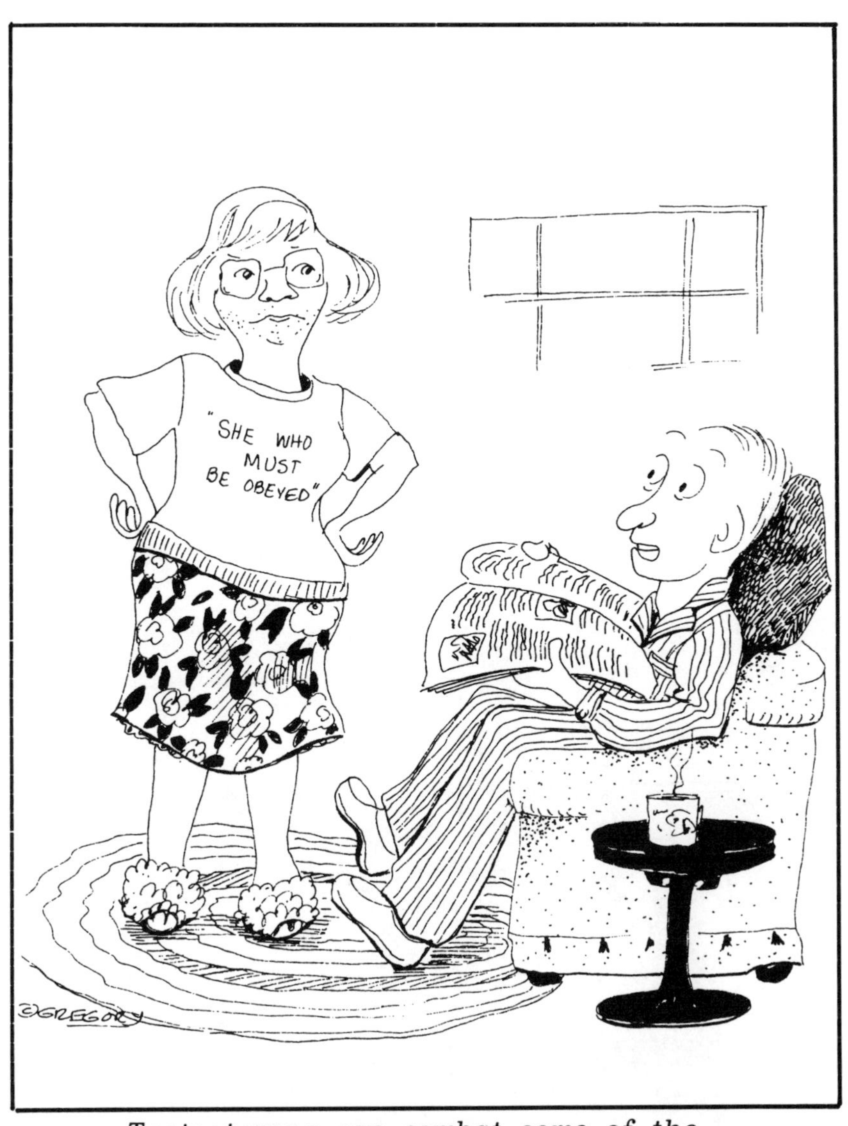

Testosterone can combat some of the side effects of menopause. As a bonus, that beard and deep voice will give you a new air of authority.

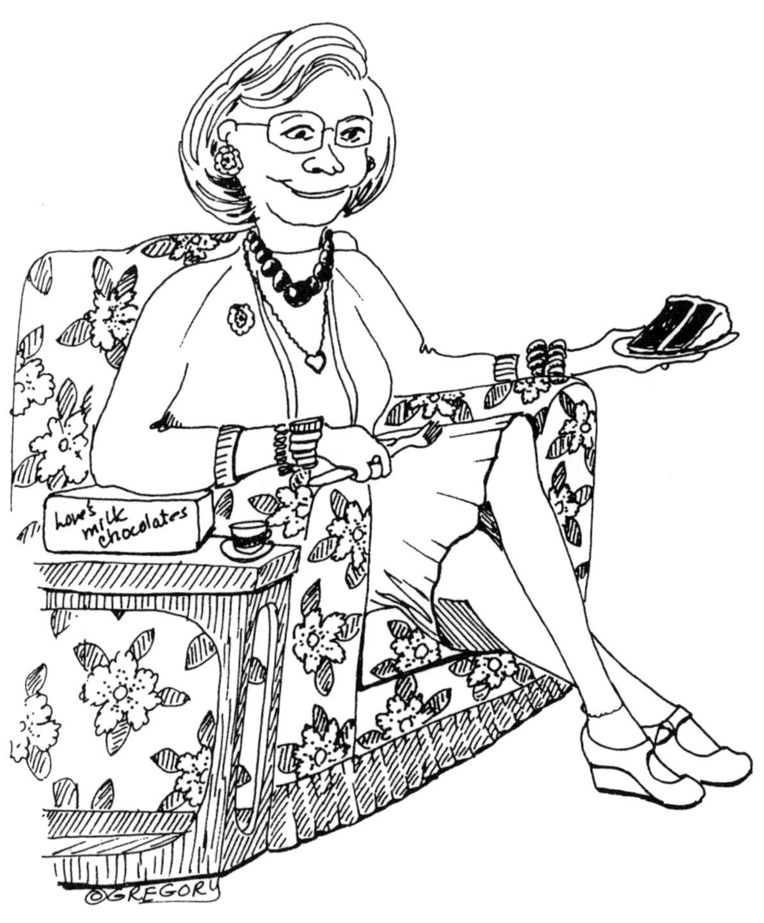

Love's milk chocolates
©GREGORY

METAMORPHOSIS

*A signal here, a symptom there
    and suddenly, we've changed.
As season follows season,
    our lives are rearranged.*

*Grief for our lost springtime
    becomes a new companion.
The Generation Gap becomes
    Generation Canyon.*

*Wintry sidewalks, slippery floors,
    become a source of grumbles.
Sticks and stones may break our bones
    (and also minor tumbles).*

*Once we measured life by months,
    now let that rhythym go...
Forget the calendar and clock,
    relax and take it slow.*

*See it as a chance to shine
    and glitter like the sun!
Our fruitful life is over,
    but harvest has begun!*

WHEN ALL'S SAID & DONE

Postmenopause.   The word's a flop!
Starts with after, ends with stop!

And like a sour note of song
MEN in the middle don't belong!

Can't we coin a word that's chipper,
Brighter, nicer, cuter, flipper?

A phrase that's foolish, girlish,brave-ish,
Not quite so "one-foot-in-the-grave-ish?"

How about, as that time nears,
The there's-no-need-to-wonder years?

The afterlife, or hiphooraytime,
Over-and-done with, happy-day-time?

So let's have laughter and applause,
because...
We won't call it postmenopause!